MW00479470

# CinergE:
# Energy Healing and
# Communication for Horses

## BY CINDY BRODY

Photos by Sam Brody

**CinergE is not a substitute for Veterinary care. It is recommended that you contact your Veterinarian when concerned about the health of your horse.**

For more information, contact:

Cindy Brody

Cindy@CindyBrody.com

(845) 679-3393

Or visit Cindy on her website, at:

www.CindyBrody.com

This is dedicated to all the horses that I have been so blessed to lay my hands on. The horses have helped me to teach their owners, grooms and riders about the importance of energy, communication and healing. Together we are making a difference not only in their lives, but also in the lives of those who love them.

I also would like to thank my family for their love and support and endless hours of listening to me talk about horses.

# Contents

### CinergE: Energy Healing and Communication for Horses

When I first started doing energy work with horses a client said to me, "I've never heard of it but if it makes a difference for my horse, then I'm all for it."

The horses opened the door to so many people who had no belief in energy work by simply improving in their jobs and temperament. Relationships have been renewed with greater understanding and as a result everyone is more fulfilled.

A happy horse is a safer horse. CinergE helps to bridge better understanding between horse and rider.

CinergE is a fusion of alternative bodywork treatments designed to bring health and well being to living creatures of every kind. CinergE combines energy balancing, Reiki, muscle testing, energetic massage and animal communication to locate and treat physical imbalances that cause mental and physical stress to your horse.

Energy work is simple, very effective and easy to learn. It will enhance your horse's soundness mentally and physically. This, in turn, will increase your horses' ability to do his or her job, whether it is jumping, dressage, trail riding or a pasture ornament. CinergE will deepen your heart connection and understanding of each other.

In this manual, you'll learn how to find where your horse feels discomfort as well as how to effectively treat his pain with just a gentle loving touch.

* Energy work will help you facilitate your horse's well being; it is not a substitute for good stable management and veterinary care.

## Basic Energy Balancing Techniques
## Getting Started

Treatments usually take about an hour once your hands become accustomed to utilizing the components of CinergE. Everyone will work at his or her own pace. Some will work more quickly, some will work a little slower, and both will be equally as effective. The more you practice, the quicker your fingers will move over your horse and your intuition will awaken more with each day.

Always work with your horse when you have plenty of time. I recommend that you start by working on one component at a time. Your horse will love the new sensitivity in your fingers, so relax and enjoy the practice. Plan to have at least an hour set aside for you and your horse. By taking your time and quieting your busy mind, you will be able to feel blocked energy release in your hands.

Another frequent question is "Where should I practice with my horse?" I love when someone can hold the horse I'm working on, but in busy barns this isn't always possible. When you are working alone with your horse, you can use crossties if he is comfortable on them. You can adjust the ties so that he can hang his head down as he relaxes.

I often work on horses in their stalls and let the horses shift around a little or munch hay, but as a beginner, you really want to be able to see your horse's responses clearly. Seeing his sometimes-dramatic releases will help you to connect with the energy release sensation in your fingers. Horses love energy work, and as they release their blockages they will stretch, lick, chew and yawn. A horse that is chewing hay is still releasing, but you won't be able to see it.

**Look and See: a picture is worth a thousand words**

The first step to learning energy balancing is to simply look at and evaluate your horse. Take notes as you look him over with a careful eye.

- Is your horse in good weight?
- Does his muscle definition look tight in his neck and shoulders?
- Or does he look nice and loose and round?
- Are some muscles more developed than others?
- Does the right side of his top line match the left side?
- Is he standing evenly on all 4 feet?
- Or is he always resting a leg by not putting weight on it?
- Does he point one of his front feet?

Now have someone walk him for you.
- Is he relaxed with his head low?
- Are his hips swinging from side to side or do they look tight with no swinging motion?
- Does he swing his front legs out in front of him or does he have a short stride?

- Do his hind feet reach into the front hoof prints as he walks? Does he limp?

Now look at his body.

- Is his coat shiny?
- Does he have any cuts or scrapes?
- Next, touch your horse. Run your hands over his entire body and legs.
- Do you feel any hot or cold areas?
- Does your horse react differently when you touch different parts of his body?
- Can you feel tight muscles and tenderness?

Last, but not least…does he look happy?

- Are his ears relaxed or are they pinned back?
- Is his chin a tight knot?
- Did he switch his tail when you were running your hands over him?

- Or are his eyes soft?

- Are his ears following you as you touch him?

- Is he licking and chewing as you scan his body?

Again, record your findings. They will be very helpful as you learn to help release energetic blockages. You will see your horse's body change before your eyes. Muscles will soften, becoming less angular. His expression will soften, and he will give you a sigh of relief. When he looks at you his expression will also change, and there will be a new bond.

**Nuts And Bolts of Energy Balancing:**

**The "Flick Test" basic muscle testing**

Your fingers are your most effective tools for finding places on a horse's body where energy is blocked. Muscle testing is simple to learn, so take a deep breath and release any worries. Here's how to muscle test: hold your first two fingers up in the form of a shallow V (like a peace sign), thumb crossed over ring finger.

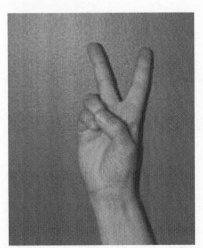

Keeping your hand in this shape, now lightly run your index finger and middle finger over the horse, using long, sweeping movements. When you come across an imbalance, your fingers will automatically pull apart.

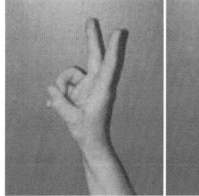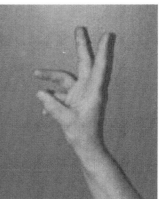

It's an involuntary flick; it marks where there is an energy imbalance. Often you'll find a tight muscle at this spot, or it may feel hot or cold. Your horse will respond by licking or chewing or even looking surprised.

The flick test is very easy to learn. Mastering it will open up a world of possibilities for you and your horse. Everybody can learn to do this test--in fact, my favorite people to teach are those who say they'll never be able to do it. What flick test success mostly requires is quieting the busyness of your mind and allowing your fingers the freedom to search for imbalances.

The flick test touch is a very light one. You're not dragging your fingers over the horse's body, you are just lightly sweeping. You are not telling your fingers to pull apart; you're allowing them to separate naturally. The more you practice, the easier your test will develop.

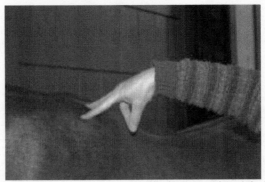

Figure 1: Lightly sweep your testing hand over your horse's body.

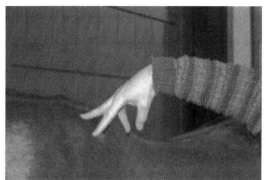

Figure 2: Your fingers will involuntarily separate when they find an imbalance.

Some student's hands will, at first, slow down over an imbalance. This marks the beginning of "getting" the flick test. If you find this keeps happening to you, try to purposely flick your finger. This will help to train your hand to do it spontaneously. You can also just practice flicking your fingers over and over again until it feels natural.

One of the greatest things about CinergE is that it can be practiced on any living creature, but I suggest someone in the learning stages limit flick test practice to people, dogs, cats and of course, your horse. I've worked on animals as varied as snakes, turtles, rabbits and cows (and I hope someday to get the chance to work on an elephant!) but it's better to practice with animals whose behavior you're familiar with.

As you're learning CinergE you can practice on house pets and human family members during quiet times, like when watching television, for example. Call your dog over and lightly scan her body with your flick test. Sometimes the flick test comes when your not focusing on it, it simply happens! We are really all "naturals" with this work. When we allow our hands the freedom to explore without questioning, they will go right to an imbalance. Human "guinea pigs" are valuable for their ability to provide verbal feedback.

## Judy's Story

Judy is a very dedicated horse person who had seen the results of CinergE techniques in a barn where she worked. She wanted to learn energy balancing in order to help her aging pony, but she was very nervous when she arrived at my weekend clinic. Her first words to me were, "I'm never going to get this. I'm not physic," and it seems that this was what she told herself over and over as the clinic progressed. "I don't feel anything," she kept lamenting.

As the class watched Judy try to learn the flick test, it was clear to all that every time she passed over an imbalance her hands would come to halt. She WAS actually getting it, and rather quickly too, but had a hard time believing it. She kept practicing and by the second day she was flicking away. "Did I do that?" she'd ask as the horse she was treating started to chew and then produced a big relaxed yawn. Her nervousness began to turn into excitement.

Monday morning I received a phone call from a very excited Judy. "It works!" she told me. "I treated my pony and he's eaten his breakfast with same enthusiasm he used to!" After breakfast he played with her other horse. Her pony was obviously feeling the best he had in a very long time, and she was thrilled!

I always tell people that when they sign up for a clinic they must leave their worries at the door. Fear and anxiety will not help you learn this work, and when you can let go of them, you'll go home with something that will potentially change your life-- and the life of every member of your family.

It takes practice to get your flick. Don't get frustrated, and don't think too hard. This work is intuitive, not cerebral! It's comparable to the art of water dousing--except that it's energy we're looking for, and it's our touch, not a forked twig, that will uncover its imbalances. Truly, everyone can learn this. You don't need a special power or a higher calling for it—just practice and an open mind.

Be especially aware of negative self-talk--it never helps any situation and will hinder your ability to learn here. Interrupt negative thought patterns with positive self-talk. "I can do this" is much more helpful and effective than "I can't get it!"

It's also important to remember that when you take a clinic, it is not a competition, don't get frustrated if other people seem to be getting it and you think that you aren't.

When I learned the flick test, I was able to get it very quickly, but I'd already been doing energy work for years. Jill, a fellow student, was working very hard to get her flick test. She

worked and worked at it--in fact she was working
way too hard.

At the end of the clinic I was thrilled with
my new knowledge, but Jill was angry--because
she couldn't get it. She could not get out of her
own head. All it takes is relaxing and trusting
your intuition. Everyone learns at his or her own
rate. Remember to keep breathing, and trust that
eventually you will get it too.

As you learn to "flick" you will find the
answers too many questions about why your horse
moves the way he moves. Most importantly, you'll
learn where your horse holds tension, in places
beyond obvious tightness and strains. Finding
these places will also reveal where your horse
compensates.

Once you find an imbalance, you can start
to treat the area. Using just a light touch, start to

gently massage a circular pattern over the spot. This is not a pushing touch, like acupressure--it's lighter, more like checking a tomato for ripeness. Watch the horse's reaction. Sometimes he'll turn and look at you. Sometimes his eyes will look sleepy. Sometimes he'll stare into space as if intensely concentrating, and then begin to lick and chew. I call these reactions "processing."

After you've worked on a spot, recheck the imbalance with your test. If the area is still out of balance, you've found an energetic puzzle. These resistant spots are usually old blockages and can represent emotional as well as physical problems.

**Energetic Puzzles**

Energetic puzzle blockages require a little bit more energy to allow them to release. I use a technique I call "point work" to facilitate this process. Here's how to do it: position your index finger, middle finger and thumb into a pyramid shape--your fingertips will form a triangle, and place them on the blockage.

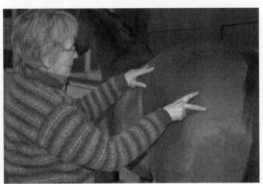

Figure 3: Many horses have energetic puzzles in their hips.

Rest your fingers on the blockage without any pressure, and simply hold them there until you feel a tingling, a pulse, or a heat release in your fingertips. Your horse will let you know when he is releasing by licking, chewing, yawning or stepping away. Sometimes you'll see his eyes start to close.

This work is very relaxing for your horse and for you as well. Remember-- as your horse releases, you should breathe and release with him. When I'm working with my regular horses, I often close my eyes, clear my mind, breath and relax. I am then more aware of my intuition and the releases of blocked energy.

## Benefits of Energy Work

Horses are extremely sensitive to touch, and this quality helps them release blocked energy very easily. Energy release helps muscles soften which increases circulation and detoxifies tissue, reducing inflammation. Soft muscles and tendons are also less prone to injury than rigid ones.

Energy work brings healing circulation to arthritic joints and also helps injuries heal more quickly. An injured horse compensates for pain by overusing and overstressing other parts of its body. When you find a horse that's tight in its right shoulder, you'll usually find that it's also tight in its left hip. Energy balancing helps minimize the strain of compensation.

I've worked with horses of all ages, shapes, sizes and jobs through the years, from foals to retired performance horses. CinergE has helped to transition horses from one career to the next.

Racehorses that come off the track have many issues, mental and physical. CinergE helps to release pain caused by track injuries and emotional traumas. Once the physical pain is relieved, the horses are able to calm down and can begin to let go of fear. With regular treatments these horses start to let go of painful memories and realize that humans can be trusted. Life on the track can be brutal for these beautiful and sensitive horses.

As any woman who's ever had a baby can attest, childbearing is a very physical experience. Broodmares suffer from maladies such as sore backs, tight hips and swollen fetlocks. CinergE helps them to stay comfortable by keeping muscles relaxed, loose and supple. A mare whose body is loose and supple is much less likely to have foaling difficulties.

An additional benefit of doing energy

balancing with broodmares is that it will give you an amazing connection to not only the mare, but her foal as well. When the foal of a routinely energy balanced mare is born, it often acts as if it's already had energetic imprinting. The foals whose mothers I've worked on often follow me around and insist on being worked on as well. They will flick my hands onto their backs just like a dog that loves to be massaged.

Energy balancing of newborn foals helps to relieve the strain of birth, supports rapid growth, and helps them weather the bumps and bruises of learning how to be a horse.

**The Reiki Ideals**

As presented by Mrs. Takata:

- ♦ Just for today, I will let go of anger.
- ♦ Just for today, I will let go of worry.
- ♦ Just for today, I will give thanks for my many blessings.

- Just for today, I will work honestly.
- Just for today, I will be kind to my neighbor and every living thing.

Reiki is the channeling of spiritually guided life-force energy. As a student learning Reiki, you will go through a series of attunements. Ancient Reiki symbols are drawn into the palms of your hands and crown chakra, which opens them to receive more life force energy. The attunements help to open up all of your chakras to receive more energy for healing, facilitating a deeper awareness of your intuition. After a Reiki attunement, you will feel more "heat" in your hands and your energetic fireball will be greatly be enhanced.

A Reiki Master is someone who has studied and mastered the 3 attunements of Reiki. It does not make them a spiritual master, although many Reiki Masters have studied many spiritual modalities and can offer spiritual guidance.

This is a short version of how Reiki has

come into being: Reiki's history goes back to Japan in the late 1800's where Dr. Miako Usui rediscovered the ancient healing symbols. In 1925 Dr. Usui passed the healing symbols to Dr. Chujiro Hayshi as a Reiki Master. In 1936 in Hawaii Mrs. Takata received her Reiki master attunement from Dr. Hayashi.

No one knows the exact origin of the Reiki symbols, but it is accepted that they are ancient symbols from Tibet, China and, some have even speculated, India.

Reiki master attunements, at one time, were very expensive and could run close to $10,000.00. Mrs. Takata thought that by making attunements expensive, Americans would respect Reiki more and that they would hold it dear.

Today, you can be attuned for somewhere around $150.00 for level 1 and 2. The Reiki Master level might be more expensive, depending on the Reiki Master you work with. You may be able to find someone who will slide his or her attunement fee.

The healing symbols have been secrets until recently, when a few Reiki teachers published them. This has caused quite a commotion in the Reiki world. Diane Stein's book *Essential Reiki* was among the first, and she wanted to share the gift with as many as possible as a way to heal the world.

Reiki attunements are a wonderful way of bringing more sensitivity to your hands. It is a simple way to treat any living creature by the simple laying on of hands. I self-treat everyday and it keeps my energy field glowing brightly. In my practice, the dogs and horses can't wait for me to place my hands gently on them. They will fling my hands on them with their noses and then close their eyes.

A Reiki healing session is very relaxing and calming. You are fully dressed for the treatment. You will be treated on a massage table or chair. Lying down is the best way to receive Reiki, although I have treated many people in chairs. There are 15 different hand positions, although the hand positions may vary with each Reiki master.

The Reiki practitioner will lightly place their hands on you, starting at your head, moving down your body all the way to your feet. You will feel the Reiki heat or energy coming from their hands, especially in places where you hold tension. Most people will have a hard time staying awake.

The Reiki practitioner does not take on their client's energy, they simply allow the energy to come through their hands. When I practice Reiki I always feel refreshed after giving a treatment.

The Reiki energy is considered an intelligent energy and will go to where it is needed.

A Reiki practitioner does not diagnose a client when we are giving a treatment. The intention is to help the client by laying our hands on them.

Reiki can be used for all family members. I love to practice on my dogs. As I lay my hands on, I allow my dog to move around. As we all know, some dogs have a hard time holding still, so I will let them move about as needed. If you have a wiggle worm, I use my intuition as to where to lay my hands. Once your dog is used to regular Reiki treatments, they will lay still for you.

Remember that, when performing Reiki, you're using a light touch. You're not pressing your hands on your client, just lightly resting them.

Horses love Reiki and will fall asleep minutes after you place your hands on them. You can treat a horse with just Reiki by starting at the their head and gradually moving your hands down the neck, shoulders, legs, back, hips and hind legs.

Allow your intuition to tell you how long to stay in any one area. Your horse will go into a deep relaxation and so will you. Practicing Reiki on your horse will sharpen all your other energetic skills.

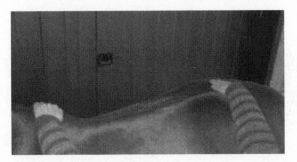

Figure 4: With one hand on the withers and one on the sacrum I run energy between the two points.

Reiki can also be used above body or long distance. Remember the fireball exercise? If you have a horse that is in pain and doesn't want you to touch his injury, you can treat by beaming your hands from above the area of concern. You can be several feet away and your horse will still feel the energy. Horses are very sensitive to energy and often times once you have done Reiki above the body, they will let you touch the injured area.

Long distance Reiki can be sent around the world. I have treated many horses that were either traveling or too far away to come in for a treatment. When I know I have a horse that is either ill or living in stress, I will send them Reiki by using the Reiki symbol for long distance healing.

Finding a Reiki Master to study with is easy and has become very commonplace in most cities. Community Colleges offer Reiki in their continuing education classes. It is very much like finding a good Doctor; ask around. Ask your chiropractor or massage therapist if they have ever worked with a Reiki practitioner. When you locate one in your area, call and ask for a telephone consultation. This is actually an interview to learn if your personalities will work together. If you're not comfortable talking on the phone with them, then you won't want to study with them or have them treat you.

There are many questions you should ask to

find the right Reiki Master for you, such as:

- How long have they been a Reiki Master?
- What kind of practice do they have?
- Are they animal lovers (always important to me)?
- Have they ever treated animals?
- What do they consider their specialty?
- How much do they charge and, if necessary, do they slide their fee?
- How far away do they live from you?
- How long have they been teaching?
- How often do they hold classes?
- Can you give me references?

Okay, now you have all the answers to all your questions. If you feel comfortable that this might be the Reiki Master for you, then make an appointment for a treatment. It is very important for you to become familiar with what a Reiki treatment can do for you and, in turn, it will help you to understand what it can do for your dog.

If for any reason you feel uncomfortable with the Reiki Master you have interviewed, keep looking and trust your intuition. You should never feel like the teacher is condescending or the all-mighty healer. We all have the ability to facilitate healing for others. The actual healer is the person who is receiving the treatment. We heal ourselves with help from practitioners; when too much ego is involved it's time to find another teacher.

Every person will have different strengths when learning CinergE. Some people might pick up the animal communication aspect more easily and some might feel a deeper connection with the hands-on aspect. As you practice, all the individual components will develop and each technique will support the other. Learning the building blocks of CinergE is very rewarding.

*Reiki A Comprehensive Guide* by Pamela Miles, is a great book for anyone who is interested in learning more about Reiki. Pamela is a Reiki Master who has been in complementary care for over thirty years. She has brought Reiki into hospitals and has been in practice since 1986.

**Above Body Work**

Using a flick test often leads me to body areas that are holding heat, which is a telltale sign of pain and inflammation. Using the tools of CinergE, I'm able to pull the heat out, facilitating swelling reduction and increased circulation.

Pulling out heat is just another tool anyone can learn. Here's a good practice for this method: rub your hands together vigorously, then stop and hold them about three inches apart. They will feel much hotter than they did before. Bring your hands further apart. Can you still feel the heat? Can feel the tingling of energy? Play with this feeling; move your hands closer together and capture the energy between them (I call this creating a fireball). Try creating a figure eight with the energy. Close your eyes and see how it feels.

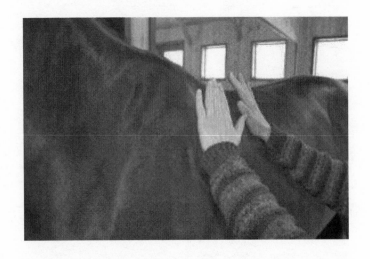

The more you practice this technique, the more sensitive your hands will become to finding imbalances.  When I first started energy balancing, I used this method as my main source of treatment. By scanning with my hands about 6 inches above the body, I could find where there was too much heat. I would then pull it out releasing inflammation. People loved the feeling of the heat release; swellings would go down and pain would disappear, all without touching.

My favorite imagery for this technique is to

see my hands as magnets. Holding my hands about three inches above a horse's body, I pull and flick the heat out. As the heat is whisked off of the horse, I visualize it going down into the earth to be cleared, up into the stars to be recharged, then instantly returned to the horse as cleansed and re-energized energy. This is the ultimate recycling.

## Sponging

People often ask me if I take on my client's imbalanced energy. The answer is an emphatic *no*. I'm also asked if I give away my energy. The answer once again is *no*. I don't take on or offer energy; I channel universal life energy. Anyone can do this; I did it for years before I had ever heard of Reiki. I do recommend a Reiki attunement for anyone who wants to help heal animals or other people.

So remember; CinergE facilitators never take on a horse's pain--we channel energy in to release blockages, so that the horse can heal itself. Our horses heal themselves with our help. Treating our horse's imbalances should not exhaust us--we are instead revitalized by the experience. As we channel energy, we are ourselves being recharged.

If you feel you need help to avoid sponging (absorbing another's energy), think of protecting yourself this way: visualize invisible cuffs on your sleeves that reflect blocked energy off of your arms. Use this, or make up your own image. Be creative--the imagery work is amazingly effective!

## Releases

Throughout the clinic, you'll hear me mention releases over and over again. Horses cannot pretend to feel relaxed, and so watching your horse release is very gratifying. Here again are the major releases you will see during a treatment: Your horse will lick, chew, yawn, and pull his jaw from side to side; he may look at you intensely (I call it the processing look) and then do a combination of releases; he may close his eyes, drop his head and relax, or he may step away from you.

If your horse stands quietly and doesn't seem to release, don't worry--it doesn't mean he's not benefiting from your touch. I've treated several horses that didn't seem to be "getting it" during their first treatment. On my second visit, they were excited to see me, and released beautifully. Sometimes horses are surprised that I can find every little sore spots. If your horse is very sore, start with short sessions so he can release little by little, he will thank you.

## Testing Progression

The first thing to do when starting to work on a horse is to balance the "fuses," three sets of key body points that represent linkages for the emotional, mental and physical energy systems. Use the flick test in order to determine whether the fuses are "in' or "out." If your fingers pull apart as they move over them, then the fuses are out of balance.

1. The Emotional Fuses

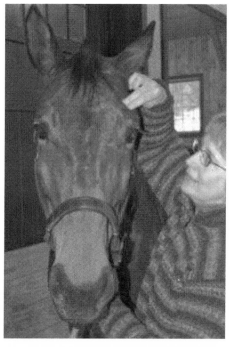

...are in the sockets over the eyes. When these fuses are out of balance it means that something is upsetting your horse. It could be something as simple as a change of stall location. It could be a change from sweet feed to pellets. It could be a training problem.

2. The Mental Fuses

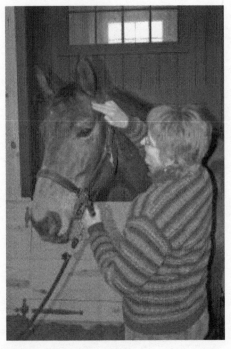

...are below the ears (the bone there looks like a V). If these fuses are out of balance, it means the horse has been through some kind of trauma. It could indicate that the horse has been abused, or has run through a fence, or has had a very bad experience.

3. The Physical Fuses

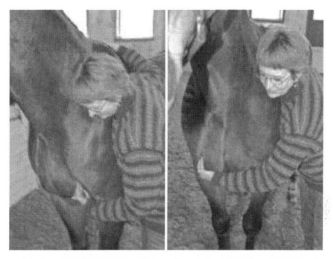

...are located on your horse's chest, in the pectoral groove. These fuses can be out for a variety of reasons. The first thing I look for is any change in hay. I look especially for moldy or dusty hay. Airborne springtime molds will also affect these fuses. If the fuses are always out I suggest a Lyme titer be drawn. Lyme disease is a tick-born illness that can cause lameness, soreness, fever, loss of appetite and personality changes. If you live in an area where ticks thrive you should be aware of how to check for, and then safely remove, ticks. If your horse has ticks always carefully check yourself and dogs as well. You could also be a host.

Imbalances in physical fuses could also indicate an upset stomach. If you find these fuses are out and your horse is a little lackluster, keep a watchful eye. Know the symptoms of colic; it could save your horses life. This manual includes a page with special instructions on using CinergE for a horse in colic.

If you think your horse is experiencing colic, call your veterinarian. Energy work can greatly help to soothe your horse, but please be sure to follow all your veterinarian's instructions. CinergE does not replace veterinarian care-- it complements it, and when used regularly can help to prevent injuries.

Colic warning aside, there's generally no need for alarm if the fuses are out of balance--it's just a signal to keep a slightly more watchful eye on your horse. Most of the time, when a fuse is returned to balance, it stays that way.

## Balancing Fuses

To bring the emotional and mental fuses back into balance, lightly rub them in a circular motion. People often ask which direction to circle in, and my answer is to use your intuition and rub in whichever way feels right. Your intention to help is the most important part of this work. It's very similar to a mother caring for a sick child--her loving intent truly helps to heal and soothe.

I balance the physical fuses with "lazy 8's." I use a light touch that moves from the left pectoral groove to the right pectoral groove in a figure-8 pattern. If these fuses have been out of balance for a while, these spots may be sore. A gentle touch is all that's necessary.

## Silky's Story

I recently worked with a 3-year-old horse named Silky who was just beginning under saddle training. When I walked into his stall to work with him for the first time, he seemed extremely nervous and frightened. When I tested him, I found that his mental fuses were way out, and his ribs were badly unbalanced as well. As I worked on Silky, I got a sudden picture of this horse rearing and running backwards.

When the rider mounted him for the first time, it had caused his tight ribs a great deal of pain. All he could think of was "I must get away," and he did, without warning, leaving his rider on the ground. Fortunately, the farm management knew he was an extraordinarily sensitive but generally good-natured animal, and realized that something could be physically wrong with him. They called me right after this incident, and after just a few treatments he calmed down.

When Silky saw me come toward his stall for his third treatment, he didn't run to the back of the stall as he had previously--he pressed against the bars, excited to see me. His ribs were no longer sore, his body wasn't holding a load of physical and emotional tension, and he was freed from pain and fear.

## Working On the Entire Body

Remember to treat the imbalances you find with a light touch. As you use your flick test, you can sometimes feel heat or cold in places where your fingers pull apart. Sometimes, the spots might even be sweaty. Keep notes and notice how these areas and your horse's reactions to your work on them change as your energy balancing skills and experience develop.

If you know your horse has been abused or is protective of his body, then use caution when working in the areas that he protects. A horse that snaps his tail when you touch his hip is in pain. Always place a hand below his hip or behind his knee so that you can feel it if he lifts his leg or goes to kick. Kicking is a knee jerk reaction; always be aware of where your body is in relationship to your horses, for safety's sake.

## Forehead

After you've balanced the fuses, you can begin to flick test the horse's entire body, beginning with his head. Check the poll, atlas, and axis areas. If a horse is out of balance in these spots, they will be very sore and some horses may resist even your flick test. If a horse is ear-shy or hard to bridle, don't start with the poll.

I never start a treatment with a struggle, so if I do find soreness in the poll area or the horse is fearful, I save the area for last. This holds true for any area that makes your horse reactive. I will come back to the area after completing the rest of the body. The horse will be much more relaxed at this point and will understand that I can help him feel better.

If the horse is still reactive, I will do above-bodywork from the distance of a few feet. He will feel the energy, and it will be effective in helping him relax the area. I will see, in my minds eye, the imbalance being released. Often, the next time I treat a protected area the horse will be less reactive. Remember, our horses have had these tender areas for a long while; it may take time to release the fear surrounding the area.

## Neck

Start at the top of the neck beneath the poll, and work your flick test down to find imbalances here. Again, your horse may react strongly here, especially if you discover an old imbalance, so save releasing the area for last. Many formerly raced Thoroughbreds have very rope-like neck musculature. The energy work really helps to relax and release these kinds of tight and over-used neck muscles. The results are immediately noticeable.

## Shoulder

Start testing at the top of shoulder and work

down. I often find many imbalances in the scapula area, especially if the rider habitually places the saddle too far forward. Unfortunately, this is all too often the case. When the saddle is too far forward, the scapula hits against it with every stride. OUCH! Horses can't move naturally with an ill-fitting saddle and those with imbalanced scapulas are often very short of stride.

As you flick test your way down the shoulder, you'll probably find many old imbalances. The point work is wonderful for puzzles in this area. Remember--imbalanced shoulders equal imbalanced legs!

## Front legs

Stand to the side of the leg facing forward. In this position you are out of the way if your horse swings his leg forward. I always position myself to be out of the way of moving limbs. A fly can cause a horse to move forward without notice. Always balance legs from the side.

Start using your flick test at the top of the leg and work downward, scanning from outside to the inside. Flesh is thin over the bones here, so treat all of a horse's legs with just a light, circular touch.

I always use the point work when I come to the joints. When you do this, you'll see great releases. Do not be alarmed if you discover that your horse's joints are completely out of balance. These body parts are easily affected by hard footing, mud, or time spent standing in a stall. Once you balance them on a regular basis, you'll see that they'll stay in balance for longer and longer spans of time.

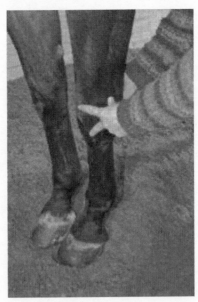

Figure 5 Point work on joints is very soothing for arthritis.

Imbalances can also alert you to structural

weaknesses--and areas that are chronically out of balance will really benefit from regular care. Remember, this work does not replace vet care; if you have a gut-level feeling that something's wrong, call your vet.

## Spine

Okay, here I go again. An ill-fitting saddle can literally cripple your horse. A horse's back pain is usually a result of a poor saddle fit. Your horse can end up with a permanently injured back from being ridden in a saddle that fits rider but not horse. "Kissing vertebrae" is a rather sweet name for a very sour injury: permanently damaged ligaments caused by bad saddle fit. It is a very sad day for the owner of a horse that gets diagnosed with this condition.

To begin treating the spine, start at the withers and work your way towards the tail. Like the legs, just a light touch is needed here--you do not need to use a lot of pressure to balance this area.

After completing work on the spine, go back and start to test both sides of it once again. You can do this by spreading out your peace sign (separating you index finger and middle finger) to straddle the spine lengthwise. Start your flick test at the withers and work down toward the tail. When you find imbalances, use the point work to release them.

## Hips

Start your flick test at the top of the hip. You can use the point work and the above bodywork if you find tight and sore muscles in this area, taking note of their location so that when you've finished balancing them, you'll be able to go back and massage them.

I like to rub arnica gel into tight, painful

muscles; Sore No More is a great product as well as Equine Remedies. I love using natural products that won't burn or blister the horse's skin. If a product comes with a warning to wear gloves, I only use it if the natural remedies need help.

## Hind Legs

Hind legs are balanced similarly to the front ones. Stand facing forward to the side of the leg. Anchor the hand you're not testing with to the hip so you will be able to move if your horse moves.

Start at the gaskin, and work your way down the leg, using your flick to test, with a light circular touch to clear the area. Remember to use just a light touch. Be careful here: a sudden rush of energy to the lower joints can feel like a tingle or a buzz to your horse, and can surprise or startle him.

I've seen the sweetest horses jerk their leg in surprise when I've started to run energy. An energy surge into an imbalanced stifle or hock might cause him to move quickly and unexpectedly (this usually only happens the first time they feel this). Note any heat in joints as you work with this area. Again, it's good to keep track of your findings!

**Ribs**

Ribs can be out of balance and sore from a slip or fall, but again, ill-fitting saddles will imbalance them enough to turn a sweet horse into a bucking bronco under saddle. Ribs and back pain go hand in hand, and once the ribs are relieved, the back will begin to feel better immediately. Please check your saddle fit. If you're not sure how to tell if it fits correctly, call an expert.

A horse that kicks when a blanket is dragged over its sides probably has a rib issue.

The same goes for a horse that kicks at you when you groom the flesh over his ribs. Run your flick test across the ribs, and your fingers will flick in places where your horse has ribs out that are out of balance. When the ribs are out, they are very painful to your horse, so make sure to treat this area with a light, careful touch. If your horse has been displaying the sore rib symptoms mentioned above, you will definitely need to do the point work as well.

## Tail

At the end of the treatment I pull the horse's tail to help carry the energy all the way down his spine. Most horses love this, but I've have had a few say, "No, I don't think I would like that." A horse may say no by pinning his tail tightly between his buttock cheeks. If he doesn't release his tail when I gently begin to tug at it, I don't force the issue. If your horse resists the tail pull, you can just massage under the tail dock. This is another effective way to help bring the energy through.

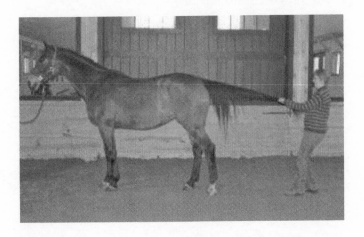

After you've completed the treatment, you should go back and re-scan your horse. If there are still any imbalances, use the point work to clear them.

Finally, I want you to take note of your horse's condition and disposition (remember the journal I mentioned at the beginning?). This assessment will be much like the one you did prior to working on him. Ask yourself these questions:

Is he relaxed? Does he look happy? Is he placing equal weight on all four of his feet?

## Post-Treatment Care for Your Horse

Water is an important part of post energy work processing, so make sure your horse has plenty of it. I've had people tell me they filled the bucket and went into the house only to come out half-hour later to find the bucket drained. Keep an eye on your horse's water intake.

It's always a good idea to hand-walk your horse for about twenty minutes after energy work. Walking will help him become used to his new balance, as well as enable him to hold the treatment longer. If you can't walk him, turn out is a good alternative, but does not replace a purposeful walk.

I always request that a horse not be ridden or worked on the day following a first-ever session. Depending on a horse's degree of imbalance and discomfort, I may even ask that he be rested longer, and injured horses always need a few days to a week off to heal. If your back is out, how long does it take *you* to feel better? The same goes for your horse.

## Post-Treatment Care for Yourself

You need care too after working with your horse's energy! Drink lots of water following a session. Water flushes your system and enhances your energy--helping you to be a better channel.

Wash your hands when you're finished treating your horse--it helps to ground you. A good post-treatment hand washing routine is to visualize the dirt and imbalances going down the drain; doing this will also help to keep you from sponging.

**When should I treat my horse, and what about working on my friend's horses?**

It is always best to get a complete history of the horse you're treating. Is he going to show or work hard the next day? If so, I'd suggest you wait until the horse is guaranteed a day off when you treat them for the first time. If a horse is really tight they will need a day to process the changes.

Many horses have been out of balance for a long time; they will need processing time. CinergE continues to process 24 to 48 hours after a treatment as the horse continues to release and relax. A horse that is very tight or nervous will benefit from a series of treatments before he shows. CinergE works on an emotional as well as a physical level. A horse that is allowed to release without stress will be very grateful to you and your relationship will grow. There are some exceptions to these rules, however.

- If you treat the horse regularly, he will actually enjoy being tweaked at a show, especially if he's a little sore. He'll be comfortable with the energy work and will be soothed by it.

- If you know the horse gets regular massage or chiropractic he will enjoy your treatments. Massage and chiropractic are different forms of energy work.

- Use and trust your intuition. If it's *your* horse and you're at a show and your intuition says wait until later, then you should wait. Trust your intuition. The more you trust and use it, the stronger it will get.

CinergE helps horses that have been through abuse by helping to unravel emotional scars and purge bad memories. I work with many horses that have been mistreated--in fact; some people have referred to me as their horse's therapist. When you listen to your horses body language and respect what he's telling you with his eyes, ears, tail and legs, you won't need a therapist. You will be in tune to his needs and your relationship will grow.

## Animal Communication

Most people believe that only a chosen few can engage in nonverbal communication with animals, but fortunately, this is simply not true. Anyone who loves animals and wants to learn to help them can easily learn energy balancing and communication as well. Everyone has the ability to communicate with his or her pets; in fact, most people already do it, whether they realize it or not. If you love massaging your pet, you are already doing energy work. When you ask your dog if he's hungry and understand his response, you're already communicating.

Trust was a key step in developing my communication abilities--once I became able to trust what I was hearing, my skills grew. Horses tell me all sorts of things, but some of the most valuable, from an owner's point of view, are the reasons they sometimes misbehave. Frequently, these reasons are easily overlooked things such as rider position, ill-fitting saddles, or a job that doesn't agree with them. Horses are honest and very heartfelt--they love to feel successful just as riders do.

Animal relationships get into trouble when the communication is lacking, just like human relationships do. My work helps to bridge the communication gap.

## Legend's Story

Legend is a 16 year-old bay thoroughbred that was a hunt horse for hire before meeting Karen, his present owner. Various riders rented him by the day to gallop through fields, jump walls, and keep up with the hounds. His former owners called him high strung and spooky, and felt they had to sedate him under saddle to "keep him quiet."

"She saved me," Legend said, the very first time I spoke with him. He was looking straight at Karen. And then he told me about his life as a hunter for hire. He said he was often so tired he couldn't feel his feet, and wanted nothing more than to stop and rest. They (his former owners) laughed at him, he said, and called him names.

Fortunately, Legend did more than just tell me what his life had been like before--he was able to share his feelings with me about the things he loved about Karen as well as things Karen needed to know to gain his trust. In Legend's former life, he was drugged and uncomfortable. When Legend told me "She saved me," Karen and I had tears in our eyes. Karen's love and patience gave Legend a new lease on life.

Legend's now able to event and hunt without tranquilizers. He and Karen have won many ribbons, but more than that, they've become a mutually supportive team: they've learned to share the kind of trust that's enabled them to take each other to new training highs.

I have seen many horse/rider relationships grow with the help of communication. So many horses are misunderstood; many "difficult" horses are actually suffering from chronic pain. In his former career, unskilled riders often rode Legend in the wrong saddle. Compounding his problems were high withers; most saddles pinched and rubbed them agonizingly. Can you imagine trying to run wearing sneakers that are a size too small? Now can you imagine running wearing sneakers a size too small AND trying to balance a lopsided package on your back? No wonder Legend had to be drugged to be able to be ridden. Pain will make a high-strung horse even higher strung, because horses will run from their pain.

Most of the sore-backed horses I work with have been ridden with saddles that don't fit. The problem often starts with a newly purchased saddle and a newly purchased horse. As the horse enters a training program, they will develop muscles and bulk. Unfortunately, the new saddle can become too tight fitting and can start to irritate the withers and back. Always look for back pain when your equine friend starts demonstrating behaviors you don't understand. Back pain is a leading cause of refusal to go forward in all disciplines.

If your horse is acting out, you can listen--
he will tell you why.

You can also speak to him--and he will hear you.

**Mental Postcards**

**Solomon's Story**

Solomon, an ultra sensitive Clydesdale/
Thoroughbred gelding is an excellent
communicator who often tells of events in the hunt
field. When I arrived one winter day to treat him,
the first thing he said to me was, "She's gone." As I
worked on him, he just kept repeating this phrase,

over and over again. After the treatment, a rider told me Solomon's owner was indeed away, out of town to spend Christmas with her family. Solomon had been left in the care of people who loved him, but he couldn't help missing her.

Horses become very attached to their owners, but they don't need to suffer when we're away; we can ease separation by sending them what I call "mental post cards." Mental postcards are simply a projection of positive energy that can be sent to any being. Here's how to do it: find a quiet spot to sit, and then close your eyes and tune into your horse. Start by thinking about what he's doing. Is he turned out? Is he eating? What is he thinking? Then, begin thinking about simply sending your love in the form of mental pictures. For example, think of some image with personal meaning for you--it can be a memory of a tender moment with your horse, such as a vision of him surrounded by a glowing red heart. There is no right or wrong way to do this--just keep playing with it until you come up with something that projects your love for him.

A postcard can also be a prayer, a meditation or just a kind thought. Studies performed in hospitals have shown that people who are prayed for heal more quickly, and with fewer complications than those who are not. Imagery work is very powerful, and horses are amazing receivers of this type of energy.

Sending positive thoughts to your horse helps to sooth nervousness about your return. If you are planning a trip, warn your horse in advance--just mentally tell him you're going to be away and that you will be coming home.

**Duffin's Story**

Joni and Duffin are a very connected horse and rider pair who had to separate for 3 months when Joan went to California to care for her mother, who had grown ill.

At the time, Duffin had suffered an injury and was confined to his stall. He was used to regular turn out and Joan was worried that the lack of this AND the loss of her company would make him miserable. So every day she was away, Joan sent Duffin a mental postcard, complete with plenty of assurances that she'd soon be coming home. Amazingly, Duffin maintained a wonderful attitude during this difficult period. It was because he knew his best friend was coming home.

**Trust what you hear!**

People often ask me questions like "if my horse can tell you where he hurts can he also tell you if he's happy?" The answer is yes.

I often just start a conversation with my equine clients by asking them four basic questions:

- Do you like your food? (All animals are food motivated and are always very comfortable talking about this subject!)
- Do you like where you live?
- What's your favorite thing to do?
- What don't you like to do?

The answers come in a variety of ways. Sometimes it appears in vivid pictures. Sometimes the pictures are just quick flashes, like snapshots. Sometimes I feel their feelings: it's actually as if my heart feels what they do. If the feeling is joy, I feel lightness. If it's fear, I feel unrest. If it's sad, I feel tears and can even get a lump in my throat. I trust my feelings and rely on them. Sometimes I don't understand what the horse is saying, but whether I "get it" or I don't, I still tell the owner what I'm hearing. If the feeling is important enough to the horse, the picture or thought will keep repeating, as if they're trying to help me figure it out. The owner usually knows exactly what their horse is talking about, even if I do not.

Remember; the more you practice, the more effective you will be. Another way to practice is to simply speak to your horse. It can be something as simple as "Are you having a nice day?" He may say, "Yes, but the flies are bothering me." This really helps to open the door to communication.

Forgive me for once again repeating myself: animal communication does not require a special gift. Animal lovers already talk to their pets, and their pets already talk back. You know how your animals feel much of the time, and as you develop your communication skills, you will know more. As you practice, you'll become more attuned to your horse's thoughts and feelings and will be able to experience a new kind of closeness.

## Bogart's Story

Gail and Rich own a retired school horse named Bogart who lives with two other horses on 37 rolling acres of pasture. It's a restful, peaceful place that's the perfect reward for a horse that's taught so many people so many things.

When Bogart started to look a little stiff in his hips, Gail requested that I do a CinergE treatment with him. As I worked on Bogart, Gail asked if I'd talk to him, and question him specifically to see if he was happy with his life on the farm. Her request was a bit tentative--she knew the energy work and its ability to facilitate healing, but had voiced reservation about animal communication.

How this horse could not be thrilled to live in such a beautiful setting, I thought! But when I asked Bogart how he liked his home, his answer wasn't as enthusiastic as I'd thought it would be. "I love it," he said, "except for...when the boys come in the barn with the white rope."

When I relayed this to Gail she was a bit skeptical...and indignant. "My boys don't come down to the barn and they wouldn't ever do anything with a rope!" she said. I told her I could be mistaken about the horse's reply, but nonetheless, the picture I'd gotten from him was extremely clear--there was a white rope and there were boys.

I finished my treatment and left. Later that night I got a phone call from Gail. She'd asked the boys during dinner if they'd been down at the barn. They said they had, because their father had asked them to give the horses some hay. They'd thrown the hay in a pile, but Bogart kept chasing the other horses away from it. The oldest boy grabbed a white lunge line that was hanging on the wall and started throwing it at Bogart to get him to stop.

Gail was amazed, but not too amazed to tell her sons this: "Bogart told Cindy he doesn't like when you do that. So don't!"

If you develop your ability to listen, you'll be able to "talk" to any kind of living creature, just quiet your mind and trust   At first, it's often easier to start learning to communicate with animals other than our own--we're so closely connected with our own creatures, we're sometimes uncertain if we are hearing them or just our own voices.

Practice on many animals. It's fun to practice on dogs and cats...or even other kinds of creatures. You'll be surprised to hear what your friend's pets have to say!

**The Turtle's Story**

This is one of my favorite stories. All creatures'
great and small have a voice.

I was with my husband at a school reunion
when the hostess asked me what I did for a living.
When I told her about my work with animal
communication, she asked if I had ever talked to a
turtle. I said I had not. She asked if I would talk to
hers. Sure, I said. She told me to follow her and
preceded to lead me to the guestroom, where she
reached under the bed and produced a turtle
covered with dust bunnies. She blew off the dust
and handed him to me. He was a beautiful turtle
with just three legs.

When I looked at him he said, "I almost
died." I told the hostess, and she said he must have
been speaking of his recent amputation.

I asked him if he liked living in an

apartment instead of the woods, and the turtle gave a confusing reply: "Oh yes," he said. "I get food here, that I'd never get in the woods." At that time, I had an image of cheese; and something orange, which made no sense to me.

Trusting my intuition I told the owner what he had said. When she heard that about his dietary delights, she ran for the kitchen. "He loves cottage cheese and cantaloupe," she said excitedly, and then put him in his aquarium and gave him just that. He ate it ravenously. He hadn't eaten in almost three weeks, she told me, and she had been very worried about him.

She still has the turtle today. They've lived together now for 15 years.

## Basics for Treating Colic

- *Never Ignore Your Horse's Symptoms!*
- *Listen to Your Horse and Listen to Your Instincts.*
- **Very Important**: *Call Your Veterinarian! Let Him/Her Know Your Horse Is Colicky. They Will Either Give You Advice Or Decide To Come Check Your Horse Out. Your Vet Will Appreciate Being Alerted That You May Need Them Later.*

### Testing Progression for a Horse in Colic

### Balance Fuses

1. The emotional fuses are in the socket above the eyes. With a light touch, move your fingertips in a circular motion.

2. The mental fuses are below the ears (the bone below them is in the shape of a V). With a light touch, move your fingertips in a circular motion. People often ask which direction to rub the circles, and my answer is to use your intuition and do it the way that feels right to you.

3. The physical fuses are on your horse's chest. I move my fingers in a figure eight pattern, going to the left over the pectoral muscles.

4. Massage ears. Begin at the base and work up to the tip. Start with light pressure and increase

gradually to medium pressure. If your horse is ear-shy, skip this part. Now is not the time to teach him it's okay to have his ears massaged.

5. Massage coronary bands. Start from the outside and massage to center. Once you get to the center, start again, going from the inside to the middle.

6. Do all 4 feet, exercising caution, because these points may be sore. Do not get kicked!

7. Belly rub. Use a circular motion to massage inside the right hind leg up into the belly. BE VERY CAREFUL. If your horse is in pain or is not used to you rubbing his belly, he may kick. Please practice this on your healthy horse to acclimate him to having his stomach touched. This technique greatly helps put the belly at ease and most colicky horses will let you do it. Always keep your free hand on the outside of the hip. If your horse goes to kick, you will be able

to push off of him and get out of the way.

8. Rectal rub. Massage inside the right butt cheek, right next to the rectum. Start light, (testing a tomato for ripeness) and then go to medium pressure (kneading bread). This will often help him to release gas. I've seen horses release virtual hot air balloons of gas doing this. Again, practice this technique before you ever have to use it to get your horse used to being touched.

**Make some time to practice these techniques in a relaxed, non-emergency situation.**

There's nothing worse than watching your horse suffer. I've seen horses die because the vet wasn't called soon enough, or an owner overlooked symptoms. Use your intuition. If something doesn't seem right, do not hesitate to get professional help

## Closing Statement

Now you have the CinergE building blocks in your tool belt. It is important to remember that no equestrian program in complete with out a good stable management program. When we work together as a team we can change the way not only the way we relate to our horses but also the world.

The more you practice the more comfortable you will become with your new CinergE skills. So get out there and start flicking away! Your horse will thank you.

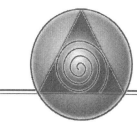

Cinerg

**Cindy Brody**

Reiki Master, Energy

Performance Body Works

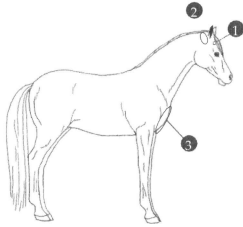

# Energetic Balancing of the Fuses for Horses

1. Emotional fuses
2. Mental fuses
3. Physical fuses

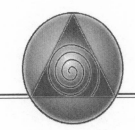

**Cinerg**

**Cindy Brody**
Reiki Master, Energy

Performance Body Works

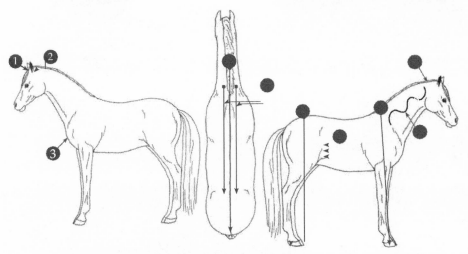

# Energetic Test Progression

1. Emotional fuse
2. Mental fuse    } Light Circular Touch
3. Physical fuse
4. Test down spine/treat
5. Place fingers either side of spine and test from neck to hips
6. Neck
7. Test ribs from shoulder to waist
8. Test shoulders to toes
9. Test hips to toes
10. Test skull

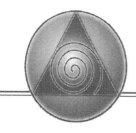

**Cinerg**

**Cindy Brody**
Reiki Master, Energy
Performance Body Works

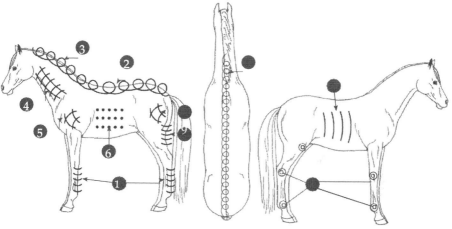

# Energetic Massage Progression

All massage stokes are gentle & light.

1. Circles over each vertebrae
2. Circular massage either side of spine
3. Circles down neck & scapula
4. Hand over hand massage
5. Hand over hand massage
6. Point work
7. Follow ribs with fingertips
8. Massage hamstrings
9. Massage hips
10. Cover joints. Run energy
11. Lift legs. Wiggle tendons.

Hamstrings & tendons wiggle from side to side

○ Cover joints run energy

••••• Point work

ℓℓℓℓ Circles over neck, back & hips

Hand over hand lower neck, shoulder & hip

## Testimonials

"Cindy Brody treats my horses regularly with CinergE body work. Her treatments are a critical part of the program that keep my horses happy and competitive. CinergE helps to prevent injuries, and when an injury does occur, it speeds the recovery and aids the horse's mental well-being. Without CinergE's support, we wouldn't be going to Devon!"

Allison K.

USDF Silver Medalist, 1997 and 1998, NAYRC,

Developing Rider list for USET

---

"Cindy manages to provide a very nourishing climate in which to learn. People took emotional risks to reveal themselves to each other and that's because she made everyone comfortable. All I can say is more, more!!"

Mary Lynne Hansen-Hise, CinergE student

# Suggested Reading

*Horse Anatomy: A Coloring Atlas* by Robert A Kainer DVM.

This is a great book on equine anatomy.     It is a must read for anyone interested in    doing bodywork.

*Reiki A Comprehensive Guide* by Pamela Miles

Notes:

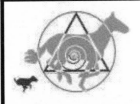

## About the Author

Cindy Brody is a Reiki Master and the originator of CinergE, an energetic healing modality that can be applied to all living beings. Utilizing a combination of energy balancing and intuition, CinergE helps to remove energy blockages that can cause stress, helping to prevent injury and ease pain.

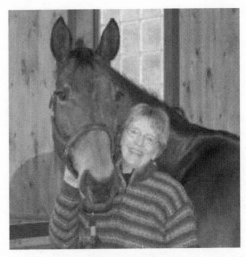

**Cindy Brody and Grace**

Cindy has been practicing CinergE for over 30 years with both people and animals. Cindy has a busy horse practice in New York's Hudson Valley and in Wellington, Florida. She also maintains an office in Woodstock, New York, where she works with people as well as dogs.

Cindy Brody is available for personal sessions, small group clinics and talks.

To contact Cindy, visit her website, www.CindyBrody.com

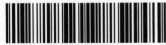

90101406R00066

Made in the USA
Middletown, DE
21 September 2018